I0441351

LIVING A HEALTHY LIFE

Eat Healthy, Be Healthy, Stay Healthy

CHANDAN SINGH

Copyright Disclaimer

ABOUT THE BOOK

In my working career, I observe so many people focus majorly on their daily job activities; hence they completely ignore health as a quest for money.

I firmly believe that health comes first because "health is wealth." If you are not healthy, you can't enjoy your wealth.

People are very busy with their working schedule, family, business, etc. They don't have time to take a look at their health.

This motivated me to write this book on the topic "Living A Healthy Life - Eat Healthy, Be Healthy, Stay Healthy"

Money is actually important, but not at the detriment of your health, because if you have millions of dollar and you are not healthy, you can not be satisfied with your million dollars.

Despite my busy work schedule, I use the tricks in the chapters of this book to keep myself fit and healthy.

DEDICATION

This book is dedicated to my mother "Laxmi Devi" because she never toils with her health.

Even at the age of 50, she decided to be healthy and she started several yoga classes. This motivated me that despite her being a busy mother of 3 children, she takes out time to do yoga in order to be healthy.

Contents

INTRODUCTION

In a busy lifestyle, it can be very hard to stay fit. Since it is important for your future to be in shape and healthy, you must learn to include healthy foods and activities in your schedule. All the chapters of this book will show you some tips on how to keep fit in a busy life.

Firstly, let's have a brief glance at some tips on how to keep fit in a busy life.

Regular exercise and eating the right foods for our body can greatly improve our health. To keep your body performing as it should, you need to keep your body moving. For a long and healthy life, we constantly have to take care of our mind, bones, and muscles. It is sad to see older people so weak and suffering from ailments caused by improper treatment of their body.

It can be challenging to find the time needed to have a healthy lifestyle. Most people are too busy with their work and families to find time to fit in a healthy lifestyle. Here are some tips on how to keep fit in a busy life.

❑ *Find Time*

One of the most popular excuses for not exercising or eating healthy is that there is not enough time during the day. If you take a look at your schedule for the week, you will surely find some gaps to fit in a few exercises. The great thing is that you only need small time frames. A quick 20-30 minutes a day can improve your health.

❑ *Find Motivation*

If you find a way to motivate yourself, you can really get into the mood to exercise and eat healthy. For some, motivation comes in the form of better feeling. For others, it could be to fit into an old pair of jeans that they have not worn in a long time. Take some time to find something that motivates you, and it will be much easier to learn how to keep fit in a busy life.

☐ Have Fun

If you follow the same old, boring practice routines, it will put you on the fast track to quitting. It's a good idea to try new activities. Instead of going to the gym, participate in sports activities or go swimming. Most of these activities can burn many calories and you won't even feel as though you are working out!

☐ Make Each Minute Count

For some, they can spend an entire hour on an exercise bike or treadmill while reading or watching TV. This is not the best way to exercise. Exercising should take you out of your comfort zone. It is better to work out hard for 30 minutes than to walk slowly on the treadmill for one hour.

☐ Get A Check Up

Before you embark on your new healthy lifestyle, it is important to seek the help of your doctor. That way, you can know your limitations when you start exercising. You want to be able to push yourself without injuring yourself in the process. Take some time to fully stretch before and after your walkouts.

Plan Ahead For Healthy Meals

Eating healthy can be hard. Everywhere you go, there is fattening and unhealthy food right at your fingertips. The best way to make sure that you eat healthy is by planning your meals ahead of time. If you work, make your lunch in the morning or the night before so that you will not be tempted into going out to lunch and getting something to eat that you will regret.

CHAPTER 1

STAYING FIT ON A TIGHT SCHEDULE

As the world gets faster and faster every day, we find less and less time for our personal needs; and one of the things we neglect is getting enough exercise in our daily routine. Some people get too tired because of their work that they would rather sleep than spend time working out thinking that they would get more tired. Some people just take it off their routine when their work load become too much for them to handle. So what can you do to stay in shape and get enough exercise even on a hectic schedule? Here are some tips on how you can squeeze it in your schedule.

You don't necessarily have to be in a gym to find a way to exercise. You can do some walking and do a lot of movement while at work. Some researchers have proven that walking and constant movement will help you with burning more than a few calories. If you want to raise the bar a bit, use the stairs at work. This burns almost as much as running and increases stamina.

Another thing you can do is squeeze in quick home exercises. You only need a few pieces of equipment, and you can get started. Since you are not at work all day, you can always do short 15-minute exercises or take an hour to walk out. I know everyone has their days off and you can use this time to take time to walk out. You can do some cardio exercises from the comfort of your own home with a treadmill or a stationary bike. You can also do weight training with some dumbbells or do some resistance training with resistance bands.

The key to staying fit is not just by getting some exercise but by also watching what you eat. If you have less time to workout, make sure that you eat healthily. This doesn't mean that you starve yourself but instead, make healthier choices. For example, instead of eating fried food, why not get the same grilled. In this way, the food has many nutrients and less fat. Make sure that you also get enough fiber in your system. Fiber helps you feel full without calories. Be sure to eat fruits and vegetables as well. We all know what they do for the body. One more important thing you should never forget to do is to drink 8 glasses of water a day. Water doesn't just keep you hydrated; it also helps with improving your metabolism. Drinking lots of water also help flush out toxins and drinking water before eating will help with making you feel full, therefore, making you eat less.

CHAPTER 2

KEEPING STABLE WEIGHT

One of the great things about losing weight is gaining more self-esteem and confidence. You stop hiding in your closet because you will finally get rid of those fats from your body and you start to feel great again about yourself. But what if the weight gains back? What are you going to do about it? Hide in the closet again?

Habitual physical activity is an absolute must for long term weight loss success. The healthiest way in which to lose weight is by using a deliberate and steady regime for both food and exercise, not by fad diets or obsessively working out. For example, a person who hasn't done hard physical exercise in years shouldn't suddenly visit the gym several times a week. Not only will the struggle to complete this regime leave you feeling demoralised, but you're far more likely to injure yourself in the process. The same goes for people who suddenly start crash dieting. Diets that restrict the daily intake of calories, or the types of food allowed can lead to a deficiency in the kinds of vitamins and nutrients that a persons body needs.

Regular exercise is very beneficial to our health. To keep our bodies at the level we want, we need to keep our bodies moving. We need to take care of our skeletal muscles, bones, and mind to achieve optimal health and longevity. We all have seen older people who are weak and seem to be suffering from a health problem that is then compounded by another, then another. So you say okay, that makes sense, but how can I fit it into my busy life? Well, here are some suggestions for you on how to improve your lifestyle.

I.   One of the main excuses people make for not exercising is that they do not have time for it. Take a look at your schedule and see where it would take half an hour within 3 to 4 days. Maybe this is a lunch break or before work. The options are available to you, but once you see the available time, you need to fit your exercise in.

II.   Another excuse that people have is as simple as lack of motivation. Take a picture of yourself and compare it to a picture taken 10 years ago. Do you see a difference in your body or how it appears? Maybe you have to realize that it's time to take action. Maybe accountability is the answer for you. You could determine if you would like to hire a coach or visit a gym. It always helps to have a partner in exercise. Maybe your spouse or friend would assist you in your training plans.

III. Many people say that they find exercise boring or prefer to do other things. Try to find something that you enjoy. Consider activities that may be fun for you, such as tennis, basketball, swimming, running on the beach or anything else you like to do. Check it out in a calorie chart and see how many calories you need in a half hour period. Do not do the same activity for each exercise. Running on the treadmill every time gets pretty boring.

IV. Use the time you train. Many people spend an hour on the treadmill watching TV or reading a book. Do the work intensively. If you have the time or energy to read a book while you are on the treadmill, do not work hard enough to make a big difference.

V.   Some older people may fear an injury. Make sure you have a thorough physical exam before starting any exercise program. An equally important step is to stretch and flex your body before and after training. Keep your joints flexible.

VI.   The work schedule of some people makes them travel always. However, this should not stop you from exercising and getting fit. Most hotels now have gyms, swimming pools and walk areas. If you want, find a mall and take a walk in the mall. During a lunch break try going for a power walk outside after being stuck in a conference room all morning.

how does a person go about losing weight in the right way?

Your body uses food as an energy source and stores surpluses as fat. This means that if you eat more than your body needs for its daily activities, you will gain weight. To lose this weight, you need to get your body to use up those fat stores. The most effective way to do this is to reduce the amount of calories you eat and increase your activity. Therefore, experts talk about weight loss in the form of sensible diet and exercise plans, and most radical methods usually work only in the short term.

Dieting can cause muscle mass to be lost, while exercise increases it. Exercise and healthy eating will help you lose more weight than dieting alone, since muscle burns more calories than fat, and because exercise speeds up your metabolism, you can cut fewer calories from your food intake, and still lose weight. Even light exercise can be of some benefit if it is done regularly. Every single time you exercise more than usual, you burn both calories and fat.

Other benefits of training include a significant reduction in the risk of developing diabetes, heart disease, osteoporosis and many other health problems with improved physical activity. Regular exercise also improves joint mobility, strength and stress levels, digestion and resistance to disease.

You should find that you are moving more easily, feeling stronger, and having a better posture.

There are lots of ways in which you can increase the amount of activity you do. Find something that is easy to do. You'll be much more likely then to fit it into your daily routine.

Other ways in which you can exercise include:

- o Try walking shorter journeys, instead of driving.
- o If taking the bus, get off a couple of stops before yours and walk that little but further.
- o Use stairs instead of the lift.
- o Try exercising at home - you can even do so during your favourite TV shows!

If you're overweight, you need to get your body to use up existing stores of fat by eating less and eating healthier options. Try lowering your calorie intake by 300-500 calories less per day. Fat contains the most calories so cut down on fatty foods.

Below are ways to reduce calorie intake without significantly changing your diet:

- Swap fizzy drinks for water
- Swap whole milk for semi-skimmed, or semi-skimmed for skimmed.
- Replace sugar in tea and coffee with sweeteners, or better still, stop altogether.
- Try eating smaller portions of your meals.
- Avoid second helpings.
- Cut out unhealthy treats and replace with a healthier alternative.
- Cut down on alcohol.

CHAPTER 3

FITNESS TIPS - EAT RIGHT

Eating well is not hard to do but to often we find ourselves saying: "I don't have the time to eat", when you neglect your healthy eating routine by not having a set mealtime or being overloaded at work.

The above statement usually follows an unhealthy snack or a huge meal because missing a meal often results in an APPETITE that craves for things that are bad for the health. You are inclined to get the highest calorie food from the menu even if you initially planned to eat healthy. Do not sacrifice your health."No time" is often cited as the reason for having an unhealthy lifestyle.

Having no time for breakfast, and yet you grab a doughnut or get some fast food, are not the smart choices, you need to take the time to plan your meals for the next day if you want to be eating well. So in spite of having the time for selecting healthy food, sometimes people start to spend money on perusing the food vending machine to curb your appetite and that is not eating well!

Staying fit involves more effort than just working out a few times a week. While it is certainly important to exercise, eating the right foods is equally important. You cannot simply exercise and continue to eat the same way you were eating before you began a fitness program-at least not if you expect to make lifestyle changes that will be beneficial to your good health. Eating healthy means more than just minimizing your intake of calories; it means eating the right kinds of foods in order to maintain healthy blood sugar and cholesterol levels.

Our society's predilection to eating in fast food restaurants instead of home-cooked meals, and preferring instant food to more wholesome food choices are known culprits to the obesity pandemic. It is undeniable that these ready-to-eat and fast food items are delicious and low-cost; unfortunately, they also are calorie-dense and have higher concentrations of sodium, saturated fat, and fast-burning carbohydrates. It is also not uncommon for these foodstuffs to contain non-nutritive and potentially harmful substances, for instance, food-grade colorings, flavor enhancers, and artificial preservatives. Apart from adding excess pounds, these convenience foods can put you at higher risk for lifestyle diseases such as hypercholesterolemia, diabetes, and some cancers.

One of the biggest problems that affects people in the 21st century is finding (or making) the time to eat healthy foods. Everyone seems to be on the go, and as a result there is a tendency to eat foods that are quick and easy albeit unhealthy. Sadly people do not realize until it is too late that they can actually accomplish both. One of the easiest ways to eat healthy when you have limited time is to take the free time you have and do all your cooking for the week and freeze it. If you don't have the freezer space to store meals for the entire week you can prepare meals for a few days and heat them in the microwave just as you would a high calorie fatty processed food meal.

Making healthier food choices will help you lose weight and assist in detoxification. You do not have to go on long fasting periods, or load yourself with medicines, or adhere to fad diets that can do more harm than good. What you can do instead is to start the habit of eating wholesome food choices. Instead of junk food, snack on veggies and fruits, and incorporate plant-based protein sources, such as nuts and legumes, and healthful dairy choice such as yogurt in your diet.

If your schedule causes you to be late for lunch and you have a tendency to snack, you can still eat healthy. Instead of going to the vending machine for a candy bar bring your own supply of fruits and vegetables. You can sit at your desk and work while you munch on slices of carrots and celery or slices of apples, oranges or bananas. Even if your company doesn't have a refrigerator (a rarity today) you can choose fruits and vegetables that do not require refrigeration.

give preference for food items made from whole grains, like brown bread, rather than those made with refined flours and sugars. Moreover, go for healthy oil choices instead of butter and lard, and trim off any visible fat in your meats to lower your serum cholesterol levels. Taking in uncooked fruits and vegetables is also a healthful practice as these come with antioxidants in bountiful measure compared to food items that have been cooked or processed.

Juicing is also another technique you can employ to bring you closer to your fitness goals and to get rid of harmful toxins in your body. Adherents of the juicing practice believe that nutrient absorption is often much faster when taking in the juices because the material does not stay too long in the gut since it is already in liquid form. If you do try juicing, it would be a good idea to keep some of the pulp in the juice because this can help fill you up. You have to remember though that some juices from fruits and vegetables contain more sugar than you might realize, so be sure to read up on their calorie content beforehand. There are also juicing routines which involve going on a fast for a few days, such as the Master Cleanse.

Those who follow Master Cleanse program takes a cup of laxative tea in the morning followed by six to twelve lemonade drinks throughout the day. There are no extensive studies done on the Master Cleanse program to test is efficacy or its safety, and some experts assert that the fasting component may put you at risk for dehydration and electrolyte imbalances which can be detrimental to your health. As we have said a while ago, you don't need to fast to drop the excess pounds. It is just a matter of making healthier choices.

Exercise is an important part of fitness as well, but so many people today are busy with jobs and school that they don't feel they have the time to fit in an exercise program. If you fit into that category, there are several easy ways you can fit in exercise without taking away from other things that take up your time. You may have read these exercise tips before, but they are certainly worth repeating.

* When you go shopping park your car as far away from the store as possible and walk the extra distance.

* Instead of using the elevator take the stairs.

* Incorporate your cleaning time into an exercise routine-i.e. work hard at vacuuming rather than working at a leisurely pace.

* Instead of taking your dog for a leisurely walk, make it into a brisk walk that will provide the increase in heart rate you need to make it a healthy walk.

☐ *Active Lifestyle That Keeps You Healthy*

If you want to stay healthy and fit, having an active lifestyle is very important. An active lifestyle means having the right habits. Your habits will keep you in shape for the long term. So what are some good habits that you should develop?

o *Exercise regularly.*

Exercise is one of the most important elements in your current lifestyle. No matter how busy you are, you must learn how to incorporate exercise into your busy life. Exercising doesn't mean taking a stroll in the park or playing with children. That is recreation, and doesn't count as a real work.

A real work out is intense. You need to be working so hard that you feel you can't lift that dumbbell one more time. This is called muscle failure. The idea is to stress your muscles to the point where it will respond and grow. And you can't do that just by taking a walk in your own backyard.

So how many times should you be exercising each week?

Ideally, you should exercise between 3 to 5 times each week. Notice that you don't have to exercise everyday. That is because you need to give time for your muscles to grow. Your muscles grow only when you give it enough rest.

For example, your workout can look something like this. Monday, work on your upper body. Tuesday, go for interval training (i.e. running). Wednesday, give your body a rest but go for a light run. Thursday, go for a full body workout. You must be tired after that. So take a rest on Friday. Saturday, enjoy the day with your family. On Sunday, spend some quiet time by yourself by going for a long but fairly intense run.

You can rest different parts of your body by rotating between different types of exercises. Don't stress your muscles too much. If your muscles are still feeling sore, rest those sore parts of your body. You can work on other parts of the body.

Of course, as you workout, remember to consume more proteins to help your muscle grow. Having a balanced diet is very important if you want to continue having intense workouts. The proteins will help build strength and repair muscles to prepare you for the next session.

Don't find excuses when it comes to exercising. If you promise yourself to exercise 3 times each week, then find time to workout 3 times each week. You will find that when you exercise hard, you don't really need to spend a lot of time exercising to get fit. Week by week, as you workout and eat right, you will be gaining strength and improving your metabolism.

As your metabolism increases, you will start to lose weight. That is the answer to having a truly healthy lifestyle.

CHAPTER 4

HABITS THAT KEEPS YOU HEALTHY

You need to start managing your life. Here are a few things you need for developing a healthy eating routine:

Eat Clean = Eating Well

Prepare a Healthy Schedule

Make the Right Choices even when you are not cooking, eating well can be done in a restaurant.

The better we do on our part to choose good foods and eat healthfully, the more effect it has on helping us stay well, feel good, and enjoy life".

o *FIRST: Starting a Clean Diet*

The first and foremost thing in eating well, will bring you on track to better health, is eating clean. Make it your health priority.

If you feel it is junk, your body will know it is junk.

Make sure that clean healthy food ideas are incorporated in your diet so that you do not ruin your body.

Natural Food Supplements:

Beachbody supplements offer proper cleansing of the body. Shakeology Beachbody supplements and Ultimate Reset Cleanse are natural supplements to help your body be healthy inside and outside. Cleansing is part of eating well, because your body cannot use the good nutrition if it is filled with toxins.

These Beachbody supplements help in total body renovation. Here is a list of Beachbody supplements to help your create a clean yet a healthy diet:

2-Day Fast Formula

- o Beachbody Ultimate Reset Cleanse
- o Shakeology, Meal Replacement Shake
- o Beachbody Supplements Hardcore Base Shake, Fuel Shot, M.A.X. Creatine
- o P90X Results and Recovery Formula
- o Energy and Endurance Formula
- o Beachbody Supplements Core Omega 3, Cal-Mag, Nutrition Pack
- o Beachbody Supplements ActiVit Multivitamins, Slimming Formula and Performance Formula

Eating Out Healthy:

Eating out Healthy does not mean that you have to stuff yourself with all the bad stuff. Eat clean even if you dine out, very important in eating well.

Healthy Food Ideas for eating well:

Make a healthy eating routine with the right kind of food supplements to augment the nourishment of the body while keeping the habit of eating clean intact.

☐ SECOND: Preparing a Healthy Eating Routine

A healthy eating routine does not mean that you have to turn vegan, or that organic foods are your only option. You can always add healthy snacks and still enjoy the best of health. The secret lies in healthy food ideas and in making the right decisions for always eating well.

Healthy Food Ideas that are Cheap:

Going to the grocery store and buying just salad is never wise. Healthy food ideas do not have to be expensive. You can always fill your cart with cheaper healthy food such as raw vegetables and fruits and make something good from scratch.

Make Small Nutrition Goals in Eating Well:

Have healthy food choices available that will help you eat better. Take the time to plan your healthy eating routine and focus on small nutrition goals instead of starting out big.

Adding Food Supplements to Your Routine:

If you believe that your are missing out on health due to your hectic routine, then it is necessary that you add food supplements in your diet to make up the deficiencies. As mentioned above, Beachbody Supplements have some options that can offer your body the proper nourishment and will help you towards your goal of eating well.

☐ *THIRD: Make the Right Choices Without Cooking for Hours*

One of the main reasons for not eating well is that you don't have time for cooking.

Add Fresher Foods In Diet:

A healthy food idea is adding fresh fruits and vegetables to your diet, as a meal replacement or snack.

Not only that, fresher foods are cheaper than eating out and are natural. Choose from a variety of fresh foods, or grab a freshly squeezed juice drink on your way to work to add to a eating well routine.

Grab Ready-to-go Food Supplements:

Beachbody supplements give you the benefits of eating vegetables in supplement form. Shakeology is a food supplement drink that helps with overall health and fitness. In addition, The Ultimate Cleanse detoxifies the system of all the junk you have been stuffing in the system for so long.

Refrigerate or Freeze the Foods:

Another option for eating well is to freeze or refrigerate the food. Cook a bigger batch of foods and divide the portions on daily basis.

The key is to keep it all simple yet healthy!

Even if you have no time, you can grab a snack on the go, develop a healthy eating routine, and make your health even better. Eating well is actually not that hard!

CHAPTER 5

GETTING FIT AND STAYING FIT!

Do you want to know the secret to get fit and keep fit? THERE IS NO SECRET! The reality is that there is no simple answer and that it is a lifestyle and not a quick fix to keep fit and stay. Let's explore the 7 keys to get fit and keep fit, and if you apply them, you too will benefit greatly.

a) Don't Buy Junk Food. Fit people know that if they keep junk food in their freezers, cupboards, fridge, car, or any where they store food, it will eventually land on their waist. So they don't buy any. Even buying junk food for your kids or spouse is not advised since

1) you'll likely eat some of it eventually,

2) your loved ones shouldn't be eating that junk either. It's called junk food for a reason, and

3) childhood obesity is a major problem, is on the rise, and parents are mostly in control of what their kids consume especially in the home.

Kick the chips, cookies, candy, baked goods, pre-packaged snacks and anything else that belongs in a vending machine to the curb. Replace the above with fresh fruit, veggies, nuts and other healthy whole foods snacks. Save the "junk food," for a cheat day that's out of the house and buy it in a one-time consumable quantity. Remember that the less that you reach for the junk food the less pull for it and the more that you pull for the healthy choices the stronger the pull.

b) Make Exercise a Priority. Fit people make exercise a priority. Along with keeping a job, paying the bills and going to the doctor, exercise is an important part of their lives. What I've found is that fit people put exercise before leisure time. Sure, fit people enjoy leisure, but it is scheduled around their workout time. Whether it is hiring a personal trainer, joining afitness program, or taking up some form of exercise you enjoy. They devote at least a few short hours per week to be active and you should too. Face it, the only fountain of youth that we really have is exercise, good nutrition, rest, and a positive mental attitude. Treat exercise time with the same importance that you would a business meeting or trip to the dentist or even a massage.

c) Do not over eat. fit people stop eating when they feel full. Sound simple? It is, but how many times have you stuffed yourself simply to clear your plate? Or how many times have you eaten another piece of cake despite being stuffed? These habits MUST be practice and the more you practice them the easier it gets. The next time you feel full, take it as a sign to stop eating. Yes, even if your plate isn't empty. Remember to eat slow because it takes the body 7-10 minutes to signal the brain that you are full.

d) Push yourself out of your comfort zone & let others Help. Not only do fit people make time exercise first thing in the morning, they challenge themselves during each workout. While it is easy to simply go through the motions while exercising, you're cheating your body out of great results when you don't push yourself out of your comfort zone. Exercise should make you sweat, make your muscles burn, and leave you with a feeling of accomplishment. Find ways to make each workout more challenging for yourself. For competitive people, the best way to push yourself is to exercise with a friend of similar strength. Another great way to challenge yourself is to set small attainable goals. These goals could be to push heavier weight, do more reps, sprint longer, or to do cardio at a higher intensity setting. And of course doing small group training, personal training, or a Boot Camp will give you the push you need to take it to the next level.

e) Don't binge in front of the TV. Fit people know that eating in front of the T.V. is mindless eating. When your attention is on your entertainment and not on your food, then you'll be less tuned in to what and how much ends up in your mouth. Eating in front of the T.V. is also very habit forming. Ever notice how you crave munchies just as a reflex of sitting in front of the T.V.? Eat before or after your entertainment and pay attention to what and how much goes into your mouth.

f) Keep hydrated. Fit people drink lots of water. And not just in addition to other beverages, but instead of them. Water is their main drink, while other drinks are occasional treats. Calorie-filled drinks are one of the quickest ways to consume excess calories which quickly turn into fat. Consider water your beverage of choice. Drink plenty of it each day and drink other beverages only a few times each week.

g) Find support. Fit people don't leave their motivation to chance. They know that if their personal trainer, boot camp instructor, or workout partner is waiting for them, then they are less likely to skip a workout. It is so easy to hit snooze or to talk yourself out of the gym as soon as your behind hits the couch after work. Fit people take the option of "skipping" out of the equation.

maintain mental health or stress free life.

Mental health is a state of emotional well-being or the absence of any mental disorder. It is also a person's ability to cope with the normal stresses of life and to contribute to society. Recent studies also show that the mere absence of a mental illness does not describe healthy mental health. It is only the health of the mind of the person. Therefore, a person suffering from any of these social, physical, or cultural effects on themselves may not be in an appropriate emotional state. Psychology is the study of mental health. Professional psychologists examine the behavior of the human mind to determine the type of illness a person is suffering from.

Different people have different mental health. Researchers refer to mental health as an attribute that enhances emotional well-being and the ability to live a full and aesthetic life, effectively combating change and challenges.

In order to maintain healthy mental health, many good and simple practices must be followed. Physical health is an important factor in the quality of the mind. A robust, healthy body helps maintain a healthy state of mind. Other minor factors that determine mental well-being are good eating habits, adequate sleep hours, stress-free work and innovative recreation.

Simple meals throughout the day are essential in keeping your body and mind fit. The skin must be kept clean by regular baths. In a breezy, comfortable room, a healthy sleep must be enjoyed every day. Physical exercise is a great way to maintain the balance of thoughts and actions. Exercise your muscles every day and take some time to practice the mind with meditation or relax with soothing music.

These practices help to control conflicting emotions such as worry, anger, and anxiety. Alcohol and drugs must be avoided at all costs in order to achieve a good emotional balance. Laughter is an integral part of life. Good humor creates a happy mood that keeps mental problems at bay. On the contrary, criticism can severely affect a person's mind. Courtesy and friendship show the good nature of a person and keep him stress free.

In addition, one must find happiness in what one should do, as this holds one in a beautiful pen. Contentment and pleasure in the duties contribute to the positive health of the psyche. Apart from the duties, a person should lead an active social life that can help him free himself from the hectic working hours. Helping others, finding the time, meeting friends, laughing with them, and visiting parents and relatives is a sure way to calm down.

Confidence building is another way to maintain a clean bill of health. By knowing our strengths and weaknesses, we must learn to accept them.

Financial problems are another stress causing factor. We must learn to spend for our needs alone and not for our wants. All these followed every day will keep our mind happy and hale.

CONCLUSION

Don't be tempted to skip meals as a way of losing weight. It will leave you much hungrier later on and you'll be likely to overeat to compensate. Irregular eating habits also disrupt your body's metabolism, making it harder to lose weight.

Did you know that obese people eat faster than non obese people? The reason is simple; these people are up to another serving of the foods. To help you feel full longer, chew your food slowly. Another thing you should consider about weight reduction is to never shop for food when you are starving because you will surely fill your basket with sweets and starchy foods instead of fruits and yogurt. Try also to cook healthy foods. There are recipe books providing healthy dishes.

It can be really hard trying to stay healthy in today's society. With a little bit of hard work and knowledge, you can learn how to keep fit in a busy life.

No matter how little time you have available, there are always things you can do to live a healthy lifestyle. The key is investing the time to do what is necessary to maintain fitness and healthy eating.

For best results, you should pair healthy eating with living a more active lifestyle. Brisk walking for twenty minutes, done three times a day, five times a week will already give you five hours of cardio workout in a week, which is the recommended amount of physical activity for adults.

It may take a while for you to see the results but be patient and persevere. Keep yourself motivated and you will soon see the results. Set yourself targets and celebrate as you reach each goal.

I am so sure you now have an idea on how to stay fit, please drop a comment on the review box.

REFERENCES

- Modern psychology 2001 Odufuwa Seyi
- https://www.psychologytoday.com/us/blog/ where-science-meets-the-steps/201504/4-life style-changes-will-boost-your-mental-health
- Book of balance diet (PG 71, 89, 72) 1999 Emmanuel Olugbenga
- https: //www.brunet.ca/en/advices/20-good-habits- that-can-help-you-stay-healthy
- Life coach master 1998 Amelia Sophie
- https://coach.nine.com.au/2018/06/04/13/47/ how-to-fit-exercise-into-your-schedule
- https:www.healthline.com/nutrition/maintai n-weight-loss
- Master Cleanse program

www.ingramcontent.com/pod-product-compliance
Lightning Source LLC
Chambersburg PA
CBHW070839310526
45788CB00018B/2599